Diet for the spine.

Treatment spine at home and without medication.

I0478535

Tell Osteochondrosis-Stop.

Author: Oleg Kolpakov.

Table of Content:

Author: Oleg Kolpakov.

Treatment spine at home and without medication.

Introduction and description:

Entry:

Symptoms of degenerative disc disease:

Causes of osteoarthritis:

Basic and necessary elements which must be included in the diet to support these fabrics:

Element 1.

Element 2.

Element 3.

Element 4.

Element 5.

Author: Oleg Kolpakov.

Introduction and description:

This book describes the elements necessary for the health of the spine.

Author: Oleg Kolpakov.

Because the spine is support for strong muscles.

Learn the important elements of relaxation exercises for the spine.

Get an excellent blood supply, requiring special attention.

The spine is strong and the structure of the discs, ligaments, and joints healthy.

An important flow of essential substances from food for the spine.

Author: Oleg Kolpakov.

The main elements that should be in the daily diet to ensure that you always have a healthy spirit and body.

Important link power of Spine healthy.

What products contain the elements necessary for the health of the spine?

Restore health spine disappeared and recover from degenerative disc disease.

Prevention is necessary to prevent the development of degenerative disc disease.

Author: Oleg Kolpakov.

How to help her back to fight with Osteochondrosis unaided.

   What are the methods of treatment of degenerative disc disease are now as efficient as possible?

How to help her back to fight with Osteochondrosis unaided.

Entry:

Author: Oleg Kolpakov.

Hello, dear reader. Thank you for your interest in my book.

Thank you for your confidence that you have shown a willingness to learn these recommendations for your health!

Now we will examine the main and important elements of the nutrition for spinal health.

Author: Oleg Kolpakov.

Take a rule that should be in your diet food, no matter you have bone or not!

When your body will receive these items, then it would be useful to have an impact not only on your spine but also to your overall health and well-being.

Items that are in your body with food, will actively participate in metabolism, tissue building and be part of all the hormones and enzymes that regulate all the functions of your body.

Let's make an important approach to your nutrition and select only healthy products.

Author: Oleg Kolpakov.

Remember:

Weak muscles lead to infringements, distortions, injury, stretching's, Osteochondrosis and hernia of the spine.

Strong muscles effectively protect your spine and support it in a natural position!

Our body needs at osteochondrosis:

Author: Oleg Kolpakov.

Problems with the spine appear gradually. And you about them may not even suspect until it happens a strong exacerbation.

After reading this book, begin today to strengthen their muscle corset, without waiting for weak muscles will lead you to injury with acute pain!

The bone must be strong to withstand load and maintain normal (physiological) the structure of the spine.

Muscle tissue needs adequate nutrition, vitamins, and oxygen to maintain normal tone and effective work.

Author: Oleg Kolpakov.

The muscles of the back-this are the main support for the spine.

Vessels of the spine and surrounding tissues should be healthy to always ensure the tissues with oxygen and nutrients.

Vessels add all the vitamins and nutrients to the tissues.

Nervous tissue-needs continuing support.

At constant voltage back and when infringements, nervous tissue is under constant stress, damaged and cease to function properly. That is not a question of normal impulses to muscles and internal organs.

Author: Oleg Kolpakov.

The main reason osteoarthritis-weak muscles, they cease to support the spine in its normal position, and the whole burden on the vertebrae and intervertebral discs and begins the process of destruction.

Symptoms of degenerative disc disease:

Cutting, sharp pain in the spine.

Numbness of the lower and upper limbs.

Author: Oleg Kolpakov.

Muscle spasms.
Headaches in the neck and in the temporal and parietal areas.

Are aching limbs.

A pain in the neck, with any movement.

Vertebral artery syndrome.

Dizziness, loss of consciousness.

The appearance of the colored spots before the eyes.

Pain in the heart and other organs.

Back pain.

Author: Oleg Kolpakov.

Tingling in the spine.

Dryness and peeling of the skin.

Increased or reduced sweating.

Spasm of the arteries.

Lowering the temperature of the skin of the lower limbs.

Causes of osteoarthritis:

Author: Oleg Kolpakov.

Causes of osteoarthritis can be hypothermia, sharp turns, in which shifting vertebrae, physical overload and improperly distributed the load on the spine.

Slouch.

Weak back muscles.

The curvature of the spine.

Being in an inconvenient poses for a long period of time.

Lifting weights.

A sedentary lifestyle.

Author: Oleg Kolpakov.

Metabolism in the body.
(Lacks phosphorus, calcium,
magnesium, zinc)

Negative effects on the
body, extended to the
chemicals.

Experienced infectious
disease.

Hyper/hypothermia.

Nervous shock, stress.

Hormonal background.

Falls, bruises and other types
of injuries of the spine.

Unfavorable climatic
conditions.

Author: Oleg Kolpakov.

Basic and necessary elements which must be included in the diet to support these fabrics:

First element: calcium.

Calcium is the main element that is part of the bones is actively involved in their construction.

Author: Oleg Kolpakov.

Calcium is a party to the chemical reactions during muscle reduction, without it this process is impossible.

The main sources of calcium: dairy products, dried fruits, seeds and nuts, fresh Greens.

You cannot get involved in such products.

The main feature of calcium. That he has accumulated in the body.

With the increased flow of calcium in the body, can provoke the formation of kidney stones.

Author: Oleg Kolpakov.

Need to try to get that element naturally than from drugs.

Second element: Magnesium.

Magnesium-promotes better absorption of calcium from the intestines regulates the delivery of calcium and potassium across cell membranes of the channels.

Involved in the process of muscle relaxation, as well as nourishing the nervous tissue and helps deal with stress.

Author: Oleg Kolpakov.

The bulk of the magnesium is in the bones.

The main sources of magnesium are nuts and seeds (cashews, almonds, and pumpkin seeds), green vegetables (spinach, celery, lettuce, leaf beet) and cereals (buckwheat and OAT).

Lack of magnesium this can cause periodic convulsions in small muscles and large muscles.

The third element: vitamin D.

Author: Oleg Kolpakov.

Vitamin D-is actively involved in the mineral exchange of calcium and phosphorus and is in the process of conducting impulses along nerve fibers.

Strengthens the suction from the gastrointestinal tract of zinc and iron.

Sources of **vitamin D** are fatty fish (halibut, salmon, and mackerel) and dairy products (especially cheese), egg yolk.

Vitamin D, even in the skin is formed under the influence of sunlight.

Author: Oleg Kolpakov.

Item four: fish oil.

Fish oil is the main source of Omega 3, which reduces the content of very low-density lipoprotein (LDL).

Fish oil, strengthens the walls of blood vessels and suppresses any inflammation and actively takes part in the synthesis of prostaglandins, which maintain normal nerve sensitivity fibers and participate in muscle decreases.

Omega 3 fatty acids, there are many benefits!

Author: Oleg Kolpakov.

The main sources of Omega-3 fatty fish (salmon, halibut, and mackerel), it is advisable to use 2-3 times a week).

Seafood (shrimp and scallops) and vegetable oils (linseed comes first).

Fish oil also contains fat-soluble vitamins A, E, D, k, they tend to accumulate in the body.

If you take fish oil or Omega 3, do not drink regularly, approximately two weeks intermittently.

Author: Oleg Kolpakov.

The fifth element: Fiber.

Fiber is fiber.

Fiber has excellent antitoxic properties.

Once in the intestine, it assumes all toxins and prints them, not letting them be absorbed into the bloodstream.

All the harmful substances are carried via the blood throughout the body and are delivered to the spine.

Author: Oleg Kolpakov.

They settle on the ligaments and bones, as a result, the spine gets additional harmful factor.

The main sources of fiber - fresh fruits and vegetables, all grains, legumes (lentils, beans, peas).

The sixth element: proteins.

Proteins-the basic building blocks for muscle tissue.

Author: Oleg Kolpakov.

When the muscles are fully built, the contraction and relaxation process in the norm.

While osteochondrosis, muscles on constant in constant tension.

Therefore, proteins are a very necessary support to ensure their durability, strength, and proper functioning.

Main sources of the protein- chicken breast, fish (tuna, flounder, COD), dairy

Author: Oleg Kolpakov.

products (cheese and curd), cereals, egg protein, legumes (lentils).

The seventh element: water.

Water is the main Wednesday our body in the water flow all metabolic processes, delivery, disposal and transfer of nutrients and elements.

Water, albeit in small quantities, is contained in the nucleus of each intervertebral disc, but if the loss of moisture in the kernel of the spine is formed, it will begin

Author: Oleg Kolpakov.

the process of degenerative disc disease.

Water promotes more rapid excretion of harmful substances from the body and has antitoxic properties.

Therefore, follow the drinking regime and drink more water instead of juice and soda.

Drink water constantly, when thirsty.

When there is a desire to drink, this says that you have comes dehydration and this should not be allowed.

In plain water, you can add lemon juice or sliced apples

Author: Oleg Kolpakov.

to taste pleasant and the water became saturated.

The eighth element: vitamin B 1 (thiamine).

Vitamin B-1 actively participates in the formation of the outer membranes of nerve fibers, is part of enzymes that help conduct nerve impulses to the target tissue and help maintain normal intestinal microflora.

Thiamine is contained in green leaves and vegetables, legumes, cereals there are vegetable oils and nuts.

Author: Oleg Kolpakov.

Thiamin has no properties to accumulate, so you need to compulsory and regular intake into an organism with its products.

The ninth element: vitamin E.

Vitamin E-is one of the most important antioxidants.

 Helps deliver oxygen to tissues, oxidizes free radicals that accumulate during any inflammation and eliminates them.

Author: Oleg Kolpakov.

Mostly large quantities contained in all vegetable oils, fatty varieties of fish (salmon, mackerel, halibut, separately-fish oil) and avocado.

Good accumulates in the body because it belongs to the fat soluble vitamins.

Vitamin E-need to take only courses in 2 weeks if you want to drink in the form of vitamin supplements.

Author: Oleg Kolpakov.

The tenth element: sulfur.

Sulfur is important to the proper functioning of the nervous system

Sulfur is involved in suppressing pain with any inflammation and muscle work and synthesis of hyaluronic acid.

Sulfur is found in fish (and fatty and lean), dairy products (low-fat cheese and curd), legumes (beans, peas, lentils).

Author: Oleg Kolpakov.

Prevention of osteoarthritis:

How to prevent aggravation of back and neck pain?

Engage in physical or therapeutic exercises every day.

Increase physical activity (longer walk, use the stairs).

Build up immunity (rubbing a cold towel, pouring, or

Author: Oleg Kolpakov.

immersion in cold water, cold shower).

Include in your diet with vitamin c-the simplest Ascorbic acid, lemon, cranberries, cranberry, Rosehip (this vitamin does not only need for immunity but also is involved in the synthesis of all collagen cartilage and spinal discs).

Sign up and go massage or a good massage back and neck muscles.

Critically analyze your diet and add more useful products.

A major step to solving your problems with my back

Author: Oleg Kolpakov.

should be improving your level of physical activity.

Change your lifestyle more head, often take in the fresh air on weekends does not sit at home in the winter go skiing, skating, summer run or even walk on long walks in the free clothes and sneakers.

Use the bike, instead of transportation. Do morning and evening exercises!

The more you move, the better your body is supplied with oxygen, improves blood flow, metabolism.

Physical activity greatly improves mood. During the

Author: Oleg Kolpakov.

movement of the hormone of happiness.

The more you live, the less you will have depression, flashes of anger, depressed mood and other "diseases" of modern man, who is constantly under the influence of different stresses.

Conclusion:

Remember, you have to take your health into your own hands, do not hope for someone else-hospitals, doctors, miracle pills!

Author: Oleg Kolpakov.

Only you will be able to help, and no one else! It is with this approach, you stand on a fascinating path self-healing!

Many foods are present in these examples, almost every paragraph, and thus combine several useful items!

Be sure to include in your diet all these elements and provide additional support for your spine.

Your meals always affect body condition, and different elements can operate in a positive or negative way.

Keep your body and health.

That's all I wanted to tell you about the benefits of data

Author: Oleg Kolpakov.

elements. I think you somewhat helped and shared with useful information.

Dear reader, thank you for your interest in my book.

I hope the book will be useful to you.

I wish you good health.

Best regards: *Oleg Kolpakov.*

Author: Oleg Kolpakov.

www.ingramcontent.com/pod-product-compliance
Lightning Source LLC
Chambersburg PA
CBHW041143180526
45159CB00002BB/721